HACKNEY LIBRARY SERVICES

Please return this book to any library in Hackney, on or before the last date stamped. Fines may be charged if it is late. Avoid fines by renewing the book (subject to it NOT being reserved).

Call the renewals line on 020 8356 2539

People who are over 60, under 18 or registered disabled are not charged fines.

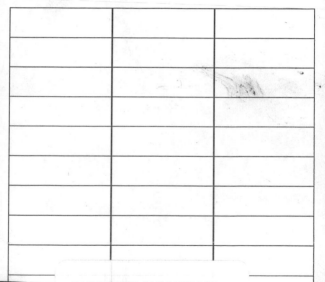

50 TIPS
TO HELP YOU
DE-STRESS

50 TIPS TO HELP YOU DE-STRESS

Copyright © Summersdale Publishers Ltd, 2013

With research by Elanor Clarke

Summersdale Publishers Ltd
46 West Street
Chichester
West Sussex
PO19 1RP
UK

www.summersdale.com

Printed and bound in China

ISBN: 978-1-84953-402-4

Substantial discounts on bulk quantities of Summersdale books are available to corporations, professional associations and other organisations. For details contact Nicky Douglas by telephone: +44 (0) 1243 756902, fax: +44 (0) 1243 786300, or email: nicky@summersdale.com.

50 TIPS
TO HELP YOU
DE-STRESS

Anna Barnes

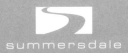
summersdale

Introduction

Stress affects people in a variety of different ways, and if left unchecked can have a very negative effect on your lifestyle. The correct amount of pressure pushes us to achieve our goals and meet deadlines, but an excess of stress can leave us feeling tired, irritable and even very unwell. The easy-to-follow tips in this book will help you to understand and combat your stress, and start you on the way to a calmer outlook. If you feel that stress is causing you too much difficulty, however, it is advised that you seek advice from your doctor.

UNDERSTANDING YOUR STRESS

Without first understanding where our stress comes from, it can be very difficult to work out strategies to combat it. These tips will help you identify, and start to deal with, your stressors.

1

Spot the symptoms of stress

Commonly, people in stressful situations will believe that they are fine, coping well, and not stressed. Perhaps this is because they believe they will look stronger if they do not admit to feeling stressed, or perhaps it is simply that they do not know the symptoms.

The stress reaction is a normal part of day-to-day life. We are under pressure to finish the project, meet the target, be sociable. But too much stress can have adverse effects, so learning to spot the symptoms is important.

Symptoms can be physical, psychological, emotional and behavioural. Some of the most common symptoms include: irritability, frequent worrying, mood swings, feeling overwhelmed, nausea, dizziness, frequent colds, aches and pains, eating too much or too little, sleeping more or less than usual, and misuse of substances such as alcohol. Websites such as Bupa or Web MD are useful for full lists of symptoms and advice, should you be concerned about your stress levels.

Understand your triggers

As individuals, we all have different needs. This also means that we have different stress factors in our lives. While there are several broad factors which would cause stress in anybody, we know ourselves best, and can work out which areas affect us the most. It may be that driving to work makes you stressed, or calling your bank. Why not try cycling to work, or talking to someone in person at the local branch of your bank? Identifying these simple triggers and making small changes is the first step to de-stressing your life.

3

Keep a diary

Once you have identified your main triggers, or as a way to help you to do this, try keeping a stress diary. Noting when things have made you feel stressed, and how stressed they make you feel on a scale of one to ten, can itself be very cathartic. However, it also provides a helpful way of showing you patterns in your stress; for example, you might always feel the most stressed at lunchtime, or waiting for the train. This in turn allows you to work on changing the situations that cause you the most stress.

4

Talk to a friend or family member

Sometimes it can be hard to know the real cause of our stress: in these cases, one of the best things you can do is speak to a good friend or a family member. If you can vocalise your concerns it may help you understand where your stress is coming from, and if the person you choose to confide in knows you well, they may be able to offer you some insight into your stress that perhaps you have not been able to see from the inside. Finally, talking is positive because the act itself is cathartic, and simply getting things off your chest can make you feel calmer and more ready for coming challenges.

5

Write down your worries

There are times for all of us when we have a few more worries than usual, be it about family, finance, career, health or any number of aspects of life. This can lead to a build-up of stress, which in turn can leave us feeling more worried. This is a vicious cycle that is best nipped in the bud. Writing your concerns down can help a great deal, especially if thoughts about unfinished tasks or unpaid bills are keeping you awake at night.

Writing worries down is a way of voicing them and helps you to think more clearly and feel more in control of your situation. Some people find the further step of destroying the piece of paper helpful, as they can see their concerns 'disappear' as they rip up, shred or burn the paper.

6

Invest in some 'me time'

We often lead very busy lives, and spend our time rushing between one task and the next both in the workplace and at home. This constant high-speed, high-pressure living can lead to high stress levels. Simply taking a little time out for yourself every so often can help to dramatically reduce stress levels and help you concentrate better, and feel more positive. At work, taking a walk in the fresh air during your break can help you feel grounded. At home, taking the time to call a friend or read a chapter of a book between tasks will help you feel more relaxed.

DE-STRESS YOUR WORK DAY

For a large proportion of adults, the workplace is the most stressful environment they find themselves in. Use these tips to help reduce workplace stress.

7

Be prepared

Work is stressful. The pressure of deadlines, meetings, phone calls and working long hours can all build up and cause us to feel very stressed. This can not only get in the way of an enjoyable, effective working life, but can also have a knock-on effect on the rest of your life, with the effects of workplace stress lasting on into the evening, and possibly the next morning.

A simple way to reduce this feeling of pressure is to plan and prepare for your work day. Pack your lunch the night before so that you are not rushing to put it together in the morning. Look up bus or train times the evening before, to ensure you know about any delays, and make a list of the tasks you wish to complete at the end of the day, so when you get to your place of work in the morning, your day is already planned out. Taking these steps will help you rush less, and give you more confidence in your workload management, which in turn will help to reduce stress levels.

8

Make a to-do list

However prepared you are, new tasks can always crop up, which is why the to-do list is such a great tool. This is something you can also use when you have lots of tasks to do at home. In any situation, it can be worrying if you have a long list of tasks that you are trying to keep track of whirling around in your head. The simple act of writing a list and crossing items off as they are done is very cathartic. Remember, you don't need to do everything on your list today; just starting the list is progress in and of itself.

9

Manage your workload

Even if you have done your best to ensure your workload is manageable, there are times when additional tasks pop up that simply cannot be ignored, or when a piece of work does not go to plan. This is when successful management of your workload is important. Knowing which tasks are more urgent, and which can wait until the next day, is the first step towards a well-managed workload. Making sure your superiors know about the situation is also important. Remember, you have the right to tell your managers that you are too busy to take on a new task without first dropping or moving one of your current jobs. And, if in doubt, return to the to-do list.

10

Learn to say 'no'

We all want to do well in our jobs, but it can be easy to fall into the habit of always accepting work and piling the pressure upon ourselves. The concept of saying 'no' to your superior when they ask you to complete a task can be a daunting one, but it is important not to worry that you will lose respect if you refuse. Those in charge understand that sometimes our workload does not permit us to take on additional tasks and responsibilities; they rely on their employees to let them know when and if they are able to do more.

Politely declining a task with the explanation that you will not be able to complete it in the time needed will not only show your boss that you are aware of your workload and limits, it will also help alleviate your stress. If you always feel you have to say 'yes' then you are left with too much work, which causes either the stress of finishing tasks late, of not completing them to the desired quality, or of having to work additional hours to complete them. This is easy to avoid, just keep an awareness of what you need to do, and say 'no' if you need to.

11

Stretch...

If you have a desk-based or sedentary job, getting up to stretch every couple of hours gives your eyes a break from the computer screen or project at hand. As well as this, it helps prevent muscular tension, which can lead to tension headaches, and it keeps the blood flowing. When our muscles are tense we become more emotionally tense, and more inclined to feel stress, so stretch that work tension away.

12

Bring a bit of nature into the office

Surprising as it may seem, research shows that having a plant on your desk can help to lower stress levels and even boost productivity. It is thought that the calming effects of nature, as well as the purifying effects of oxygen-producing foliage, are to thank for this positive reaction. Choose leafy plants rather than flowering ones as plants rich in foliage will produce more oxygen.

Avoid 'catching' stress from your colleagues

A large amount of workplace stress is so-called 'second-hand' stress. When a colleague is feeling stressed you can subconsciously 'absorb' their feelings of negativity. To avoid this, if a colleague is talking about work or personal problems, try to say something positive about the subject or offer them some advice. If they carry on, perhaps offer to go and make a hot drink to diffuse the situation, or if you cannot walk away, make sure you stay positive, and try your best not to adopt your colleague's mindset.

DE-STRESS YOUR HOME

If you are not happy and comfortable in your home, chances are you will feel stressed. Combatting stressors in our home environment can have a positive effect on many other areas of life, too.

14

De-clutter your home

A clean home helps us to keep a clear head. Most of us will know the feeling when you want to find something, be it an item of clothing, a book or a kitchen gadget, but our overflowing drawers, wardrobes and shelves stop us in our tracks. Frustrations can build in situations such as this, and cause stress.

De-cluttering our homes can help alleviate stress on various levels: with your belongings tidily in place you will not waste time getting stressed looking for them, the act of tidying can be very satisfying and the physical energy involved in de-cluttering produces serotonin – the hormone which balances mood and helps us feel happier.

15

Organise your wardrobe

Once you have de-cluttered, it is time to tackle your wardrobe. It can be stressful deciding what to wear to work in the morning, or to that special social event. This can be a stress trigger, and knowing where everything is will allow you to choose your outfits more quickly and easily, thus reducing stress.

The amount of space you have and your own preferences will help you decide how to organise your clothing, but a couple of simple suggestions would be to either divide your wardrobe into work and casual, and then into colours within those groups, or to divide it into clothing types – tops, trousers, dresses etc. Choose whatever works best for you.

Speed-clean your way to a relaxed home

Trying to keep on top of household chores when you are balancing your commitments to your job, your family and your friends can be rather daunting. If you feel it's time to take on the grime, but are overwhelmed by the size of the job, take the stress out of cleaning by tackling just one or two rooms at a time, rather than the whole job. Get the cleaning done first, then vacuum the floors, so that you are not adding to your work by making them dusty again. You don't need to clean everything in the room, just whatever is dusty or dirty, and if you wear an apron with pockets, you can carry your cleaning equipment round with you.

Finally, remember that big tasks such as cleaning the windows or the oven don't need to be done as frequently. Spread them out throughout the year to reduce the cleaning you have to do on each occasion.

Money makes the world go round

Money is the number one cause of stress outside of work stress, and the main cause of relationship breakdown in the UK. It is tempting to try to live beyond our means, as we feel, and are told through advertising, that we deserve certain material comforts. While this is a matter of opinion, what we really have to think about is whether or not we *need* that item we are craving, be it a new sofa or something as simple as a chocolate bar.

The key to controlling, and therefore de-stressing, your money situation, is to make sure you plan your spending. Having a budget may seem strange at first, but all those little things can add up, and losing your morning latte in favour of making a drink at home or the office, for example, can free up a surprising amount of cash over time. With better cash flow and fewer money worries will come lower levels of stress and higher levels of happiness.

Avoid too much TV time

Amazingly, the average person watches around four hours of television a day. When you consider how busy our lives have become, it is no wonder we find little time to do anything else if we come home from work, sit in front of the television for four hours, and then go to bed. This can add to the feeling of not having enough time and build stress.

Whilst television can be interesting and informative, watching too much can take away time you might have to talk to your loved ones or take part in a hobby, leading to greater levels of stress. Rather than just turning the television on automatically in the evening, plan what you want to watch and turn the TV off after it has finished. Alternatively, watch a favourite show online through an on-demand service. This reduces the number of hours spent in front of the screen, freeing up more time and helping you de-stress.

Computer, computer, computer

Televisions are not the only screen we should avoid too much contact with if we want to de-stress. With the rise in use of technology, many of us sit at a screen for eight hours whilst at work, only to check our personal emails and social media accounts on our laptop or tablet, and then do additional work, play games or watch catch-up TV on our home computers. All in all, we can end up spending ten or more hours per day looking at a computer screen, which causes eye strain and muscle strain in the neck. This can lead to tension headaches — a major stress factor.

Reduce your contact time with computer screens by making sure you take regular breaks at work, and try to spend time at home away from the computer as much as possible. Making time for conversations with your partner or friends or taking up a hobby can help you to get away from a screen. You will feel physically better and under less stress.

FOOD AND STRESS

We all know that food can have both positive and negative effects on our bodies. However, aside from the obvious results to do with weight loss or gain, the way you eat and drink can also affect your stress levels.

20

Balanced diet

There are foods that are said to be good for the heart, the brain and digestion – and there are foods that increase or reduce stress levels. The first thing you should try to do, though, is to get a balanced diet. Eating the right amount of calories for your age, height and sex, and ensuring you get enough proteins, fibre and vitamin-rich fruits and vegetables will give you a sound basis for general health and should improve your digestion. Eating a balanced diet puts you in the best shape to fight stress and acts as an excellent starting point for 'de-stress' nutrition.

Low GI for low-stress

GI stands for Glycaemic Index. This is a measurement of how much energy a food will give you from sugars. High-GI foods tend to be things like sweets and pastries, whilst vegetables and lean protein such as fish, skinless chicken and tofu are low GI.

A low-GI diet can have many health benefits, including aiding weight loss, and is particularly good for combatting stress. High-GI foods will cause a spike in blood sugar, which will then drop rapidly, leaving you feeling tired, irritable and hungry again. This is the perfect formula for feeling stressed. Low-GI foods, on the other hand, help keep blood sugar levels more steady, avoiding those dips and helping you feel calmer.

Eat the right kinds of fats

Although we are often told that eating a low-fat diet is healthy, certain fats are needed for optimum health. In fact, certain fats help ensure your brain and immune system function properly. Making sure you include some of these good fats in your diet can be helpful in reducing the negative effects stress can have on your body, and in helping your body to cope better with stress.

The four main types of fat are monounsaturated, polyunsaturated, saturated and trans. It is the first two types that you need in your diet, and these can be found in foods such as fish, nuts, seeds, olive oil and avocados.

Don't reach for the salt

Being stressed for long periods of time can make us crave salt, as our adrenal glands become exhausted and are unable to make adrenaline and cortisol. This results in a salt imbalance, and it can be very easy to reach for salty foods – especially as many of these foods are also fatty and comforting. Although high salt intake alone does not increase stress levels, the associated health problems such as weight gain and high blood pressure certainly do, so give the salt a wide berth. Instead, choose fruit as a snack, and prepare your meals from fresh produce as pre-packaged foods are usually very high in salt.

24

Curb your sweet tooth

When stressed, it can be easy to reach for sweet foods for the quick surge of energy they give, and for the comfort. Part of the reason people do this is that we have an inbuilt reaction to danger, known as 'fight or flight'. Our reaction has not yet evolved to catch up with our modern lifestyle, and stress is still perceived by our bodies as a reaction to being in danger. When faced with a predator, for example, we would need to stand and fight, or quickly run away, and for both of these, we would need quick-release energy.

The cortisol our bodies release in reaction to stress increases blood sugar to speed up the metabolism, and our body receives the message that it needs to consume a high-energy substance.

Our lifestyle now, however, means that our stress is more likely to be because of bills we have to pay, or meetings we have to arrange, and this reaction is unhelpful because we do not need the energy boost. To give your body the sweet taste it is craving without putting excess sugar which you will not use into your body, try chewing sugar-free gum.

25

Be ACE

High levels of stress hormones in your system can have a negative effect on your health, either by lowering your immune system, making you more prone to coughs, colds and other infections, or by over-stimulating it and provoking autoimmune illnesses and inflammation of the body. A simple way to combat these stress symptoms is to eat plenty of foods rich in the antioxidant vitamins A, C and E. These antioxidants help normalise the body and reduce inflammation, whilst boosting immunity.

Vitamin A is found in the form of retinol in products such as fish liver oil and egg yolks.

Too much retinol can be bad for the health though, so balance this with beta-carotene, found in mainly yellow and orange fruits and vegetables such as carrots, butternut squash and apricots. Vitamin C is found in good amounts in citrus fruits, broccoli, berries and tomatoes, and vitamin E is found in nuts, seeds, avocados, olive oil and wheatgerm. Adding some of these foods to your diet could make you feel healthier and happier.

Get a B-vit boost

The B vitamin group is particularly important for maintaining a healthy balance and keeping stress at bay. Amongst their other functions, B vitamins are involved in the body's control of tryptophan, a building block for serotonin. Too little tryptophan can lead to a drop of serotonin which can lead to low mood, which, in turn, can lead to very serious psychological problems. The main vitamins to pay attention to are B1, B3, B5, B6, B9 and B12, all of which can be found in a balanced diet, especially in foods such as spinach, broccoli, asparagus and liver. If you eat a lot of processed foods, or are a vegan, you may be lacking in certain B vitamins, in which case adding a B-vitamin supplement to your diet can have an excellent effect.

27

Take a caffeine break

Caffeine and other similar stimulants should be avoided as much as possible. Many of us rely on that first cup of coffee in the morning to wake us up, or a cup of tea to keep us going at midday, but these caffeinated drinks, along with cola and foods containing caffeine such as chocolate, could be having an adverse effect on your stress levels – perhaps the opposite effect to the one you intend.

Drinking a caffeinated drink can make us feel more alert because it induces the initial stages of the stress reaction, boosting cortisol production. Consuming large quantities of caffeine, however, can cause the exhaustion phase of stress. Added to this, caffeine can be very addictive, and stopping suddenly can cause withdrawal symptoms. Try cutting down slowly to no more than 300 mg of caffeine in a day – that's the equivalent of three mugs of coffee or four mugs of tea in a day. Have fun experimenting with the huge variety of herbal teas available on the market to fill the gap.

Avoid alcohol

After a hard day at work, many people will reach for a drink to help them relax. Alcohol does have an instantly calming effect, but this is negated by the depressant qualities of alcohol, and the feeling of anxiety that can be left behind once the effects wear off. Alcohol can also disturb your sleep, contrary to the popular idea of a 'nightcap'. Try to cut down your drinking as much as possible, and if you do go for a tipple, opt for a small glass of Chianti, Merlot or Cabernet Sauvignon, as the grape skins used in these wines are rich with the sleep hormone, melatonin. Do make sure it's a small one, though!

EASE STRESS WITH EXERCISE

When pressures mount up, exercise is often the first thing to go. It is easy to not find the time to keep fit, but a regular exercise routine will boost your serotonin levels, help you use up your cortisol, and let you take time off from the stresses and strains of day-to-day life.

Just walk

Walking is such a simple form of exercise, and can be incorporated into your daily life with ease. Though not as fat-busting as running or martial arts, for example, adding regular walking into your routine will help keep you fitter and healthier, and will help reduce feelings of anxiety as it will help your body produce serotonin.

Even if you lead a very busy life, walking can fit in to your routine. Try parking further from the office, taking the stairs rather than the lift, or going for a brisk fifteen-minute walk at lunchtime. It is a healthy habit to form and you will soon be reaping the benefits.

Let your troubles float away

Swimming is one of the best forms of exercise, both in terms of giving you a full-body work-out which will leave you tired for the right reasons, and in allowing you to relax and unwind. The rhythmic lap of the water with each stroke, and the focus on your technique and breathing, really make this a great way to move your mind away from the stresses of your day. Add to that the fact that floating in water is a wonderfully relaxing experience, and all part and parcel of a trip to the pool, and you've got a perfect recipe for relaxation.

31

Try t'ai chi

A 'moving meditation', t'ai chi is an ancient Chinese martial art. Unlike other martial arts, t'ai chi is non-combative, and is distinctive for its slow, precise movements. As well as helping improve posture, balance, strength and flexibility, this ancient art is meant to promote the healthy flow of energy throughout the body, and to calm the mind. Feeling focussed and relaxed can have a positive effect on your stress levels.

Give yoga a try

Yoga is an ancient form of exercise which originates from India. It has become very popular in recent years, and with good reason. Not only is yoga a gentle form of exercise, which will help you feel calmer, it can also be very beneficial in releasing stress from the body. Yoga combines movements with breathing, so that the mind is focussed on what the body is doing. This physical focus helps the mind to relax and stop thinking about the worries of the day. Why not try a class local to you, or look for tutorials online?

RELAXATION TECHNIQUES AND SELF-HYPNOSIS

One of the most common reasons people feel stressed is the inability to relax. Relaxation is both simple and complicated at the same time – these tips will help you discover ways to let yourself relax, that work for you.

33

Practise mindfulness

Mindfulness is a technique adopted from Buddhist teachings that can help you to live in the moment. This can be a great help in reducing stress. Training your mind to notice how you are feeling about situations as they arise can help you to recognise your stress triggers which, in turn, makes it easier to be mindful of when they arise and to deal with them calmly. Mindfulness also helps us learn not to go into 'autopilot' when we are doing

suitable
moment &
place.

familiar tasks, as this can be a cause of stress. Taking a shower with a mindful approach is a simple example: rather than just automatically going through the motions, notice how the water feels on your skin, the smell and texture of your body wash, the way your muscles relax with the heat. This can be a great way to start the day feeling unrushed and calm. These techniques can be applied to your whole day.

Breathe

Sometimes we find it hard to switch off after a stressful day and find ourselves in a vicious cycle which can lead to stress levels becoming ever higher. A simple way to start training your body to relax is to practise mindful deep breathing. This can be done at any time of the day, whether before bed, first thing in the morning or at your desk in the office.

The practice is simple: close your eyes and focus on your breath. Think only about your breath and the way it feels coming into your body and then out. Once you are fully aware of your breathing, try taking deeper breaths, breathing in for a count of six and then out for a count of six. Stay focussed on your breath for five minutes. Integrating this exercise into your daily routine will help you on the way to feeling more relaxed.

Progressive relaxation

Progressive relaxation is a great tool for everyday use. The theory is that if you focus intensely on each part of the body, and then let it go, you will relax more completely than if you were to simply 'try' to relax. There are many forms of progressive relaxation, some using affirmations or mantras, and some focussing on the physical.

One of the simplest methods you can use, and an easy way to introduce yourself to progressive relaxation, is to lie down on your back somewhere comfortable. Starting with your toes, and working your way slowly up your body to your head, tightly clench your muscles and hold them for five seconds, then release. The effect will be greater if you clench on your in-breath, and release on your out-breath. If you find your mind wandering, try using the mantra 'I am relaxing my toes, I can feel my toes completely relaxed', repeating for each body part. You can even find apps to help you through the process. By the end, you should feel physically and mentally relaxed.

36

Meditate

Meditation has been used by many cultures around the world for centuries. Yoga and t'ai chi are both described as 'moving meditation', showing that this practice takes many forms. You don't necessarily have to sit cross-legged and chant mantras to meditate, though you can if this is something you find helpful.

Put simply, meditation is a way of quieting your mind and allowing yourself time to be still. A good way to start, if meditation is new to you, is to sit in a comfortable position with a straight back, resting your hands palms-up in your lap. Close your eyes and focus on one of your other senses, such as your hearing. When your mind begins to wander, gently bring it back to your chosen sense. Doing this for five to ten minutes can make a huge difference to your day.

Guided meditation

As its name suggests, this is a form of meditation in which, rather than you taking the lead, someone else is guiding you. If you find sitting still with your own thoughts difficult, this could be for you. It is also more structured than self-led meditation, which can make it easier to follow.

Guided meditation may be done in a class setting, so take a look into your local natural health centres or yoga studios to see if they run classes. Alternatively, you can buy CDs of guided meditation, or download meditation tracks or apps from the Internet. However you choose to do it, this is a great way to feel relaxed quickly, and has long-lasting after-effects, helping you feel relaxed into the next day.

A HEALTHY ATTITUDE FOR LOWER STRESS

Much of why we feel stressed can be traced to how we react to stressful events or situations. Learning to adopt the right attitude and be kinder to yourself – not expecting too much and avoiding harsh self-criticism – can help your stress levels to drop.

38

Slow down

The first thing to do to help build a healthier attitude towards yourself is to simply slow down. Many of us are living our lives at an ever-faster pace, and trying to balance a whole range of commitments from work to family to relationships. This can leave us feeling stressed and frustrated when we are forced to stop, for instance when we have to queue. Combat this by taking those moments when your bus is late, or when you are stuck in traffic, to do something relaxing like deep breathing or listening to music.

Better sleep = less stress

It is hard to keep a cool head when you feel tired. Getting more good-quality sleep will help reduce your stress levels, which in turn will help you sleep better, because each action positively affects the other. The relaxation techniques described earlier in this book can help you drift off to sleep more easily. Another tip to help here is to make your bedroom a haven that you look forward to entering at the end of the day; this will also create an environment conducive to sleep and relaxation.

If you have trouble sleeping at night, try a warm milky drink or herbal tea to send you off. Alternatively, reading a book or taking a warm bath can work wonders.

Learn problem solving

Issues can mount up, and thinking about them excessively can make them seem like insurmountable problems. When we mull over a situation, we may think that we are looking for the best solution, but in fact we can be causing the stress surrounding this problem to grow, just with the action of thinking alone.

Instead of thinking over your problems, try taking positive steps to changing difficult situations. Even if you are only moving slowly towards the goal of eliminating the issue, just focussing your energy on what you can do now can have a very positive effect on your emotional health.

Use affirmations

An affirmation is a positive phrase that you use to help change negative beliefs to positive ones. Affirmations work well when written down, and when said out loud. A positive affirmation to help you change your attitude to stressful situations could be, 'I feel calm and centred' or 'I solve my problems quickly and effectively'.

It is important that the affirmation focusses on the positive outcome that you want rather than the negative possibility that you wish to avoid, and that it is written or spoken in the present. You can buy CDs of positive affirmations to listen to before sleep, or download them from the Internet, should you prefer.

42

Go green

Enjoy what the great outdoors has to offer by spending more time in your garden, local park or woods. Being in natural surroundings can bring a real sense of tranquillity. Going for a walk along the coast, through the fields or even just in your garden can improve your mood, ease muscle tension and lower blood pressure. Feeling close to nature can give you the boost you need to keep calm under pressure.

43

Love to laugh

The old adage tells us that 'laughter is the best medicine'. In many ways, this is true. Laughter helps us feel relaxed – it relieves tension and makes us feel happier, which in turn will leave us better equipped to deal with the difficult situations life might throw our way.

Try watching your favourite comedy or looking at a funny website for a bit of light relief. You could even invite some friends over for a night of funny movies and swap amusing stories.

44

Negative? What negative?

We will all experience difficult situations at some point or other in our lives, but it is how we deal with them, and not the situations themselves, that has the most impact on our stress levels. A great way to change your mind about problems is to find a positive within the negative.

This can be hard at first, especially in situations that can have quite a strong and lasting effect on your life. Even finding a small positive will make a situation easier to deal with. Perhaps you have lost your job, but the positive is that now you can retrain for the career you always wanted. Or perhaps a relationship has ended, but the positive is that you are now free to find someone more suited to you, and form a brighter future. It is not always easy to do this, but this shift in perspective can be very liberating.

Visualise

The idea of visualisation may sound 'New Age' to some, but people have been using this method for many years to help them focus and overcome difficulties. Use this simple visualisation to help you free your mind of your worries – this will be of particular help at night, when many find their worries start circling around in their heads:

If your mind is racing, looking for a solution it can't find, then tell yourself, 'I can't do anything practical to help this today. I can think about it tomorrow.' As you give your mind this message, see your worry trapped inside a colourful balloon, floating up and away, out of reach and out of mind.

DE-STRESS THERAPIES

When you feel like it is all getting too much, these therapeutic options can help take the strain away, and have the added bonus of allowing you some 'me time' to relax and reflect.

Aromatherapy for calm

Essential oils have been long used to help calm the mind and body. It is believed that inhaling the smells from essential oils affects the hypothalamus, the part of the brain that controls the glands and hormones, thereby changing a person's mood and lowering their levels of stress and anxiety.

You can use aromatherapy oils in massage oil, in the bath, for steam inhalation or as a compress. Some uplifting essential oils to try include bergamot, chamomile, lavender, neroli and rose. Some stimulating oils to try include black pepper, geranium, peppermint and rosemary.

Under pressure

Acupressure is a part of traditional Chinese medicine. Similar to acupuncture, but without the use of needles, this gentle therapy involves applying pressure to certain points on the body to promote the free flow of energy through the body. Acupressure is known to help relieve muscle tension and boost circulation.

You can go to a practitioner for acupressure (or acupuncture if you are happy with needles), or you can use simple acupressure techniques at home. There are many books available on the subject, or you can find tutorials online.

48

It's all in the reflexes

Reflexology, similarly to acupressure, uses stimulation of certain points to help the flow of energy through the body. These points are found on the feet, hands and face, but practitioners will usually use the feet as these are more sensitive, and are believed to have points that relate to every part of the body. Stimulating these points is meant to release energy blockages in the related body part, therefore facilitating the free flow of energy through that body part, and reducing illness.

Whatever the health claims, the relaxation alone will help reduce stress. For practicality, if you decide to try this on yourself, it may be easier to use your hands, and though reflexology can be self-practised, it is more relaxing to visit a reflexologist for treatment. Look up your local natural health centre for more information.

49

A good rub down

There is no denying that a good massage leaves you feeling more relaxed and ready to face new challenges. As well as promoting healthy blood flow and relaxing the muscles, being massaged gives you time to just focus on you. Look up a local massage therapist, or ask a friend or partner to give your shoulders, back or feet a calming, soothing rub. Alternatively, you can try self-massage on your hands, feet, legs or scalp.

Using aromatherapy oils such as lavender or neroli will make this experience even more calming, and help you feel more de-stressed.

50

And finally... doctor's orders

If all else fails, and stress is becoming too much of an issue for you, it is worth speaking to your doctor about it. Though complementary therapies can help a great deal, some situations need a firmer hand, and sometimes stress is a sign of more serious issues. It may be that your doctor recommends a talking therapy such as CBT (Cognitive Behavioural Therapy) or medication, to help you reduce the amount of stress in your life. Remember, the doctor is there to help you, so tell them all of your worries, and hopefully you will be feeling the benefit before long.

Notes

....
....
....
....
....
....
....
....
....
....
....
....
....
....
....
....

50 TIPS
TO HELP YOU
SLEEP WELL

Anna Barnes

50 TIPS TO HELP YOU SLEEP WELL

Anna Barnes

ISBN: 978-1-84953-401-7

Hardback

£5.99

There are times for all of us when, no matter how many sheep we have counted, falling asleep just isn't as easy as it should be. This book of simple, easy-to-follow tips provides you with the tools and techniques needed to understand your sleep patterns, and to make changes that will steer you on the path towards restful sleep.

If you're interested in finding out more about our books,
find us on Facebook at **Summersdale Publishers**
and follow us on Twitter at **@Summersdale**.

www.summersdale.com